CHECK-UP: Our NHS @ 70

D0508005

Mark Thomas

CHECK-UP:
Our NHS @ 70

OBERON BOOKS
LONDON

WWW.OBERONBOOKS.COM

First published in 2018 by Oberon Books Ltd
521 Caledonian Road, London N7 9RH
Tel: +44 (0) 20 7607 3637 / Fax: +44 (0) 20 7607 3629
e-mail: info@oberonbooks.com
www.oberonbooks.com

A catalogue record for this book is available from the British Library.

PB ISBN: 9781786825018
E ISBN: 9781786825025

Cover design © Greg Matthews
Photography © Steve Ullathorne (cover, p. 21), Jane Hobson (pp. 22-31)

Printed and bound by 4EDGE Limited, Hockley, Essex, UK.
eBook conversion by Lapiz Digital Services, India.

Visit www.oberonbooks.com to read more about all our books and to buy them.
You will also find features, author interviews and news of any author events, and you can
sign up for e-newsletters so that you're always first to hear about our new releases.

Printed on FSC accredited paper

Contents

Acknowledgements   6

Introduction, by Mark Thomas   7

Preface, by Nicolas Kent   11

Creative Team   14

In Pictures   21

CHECK-UP: Our NHS @ 70   33

Acknowledgements

Thanks go to the Wellcome Trust for their support and to everyone mentioned in this play, as well as the many others who contributed ideas and help and gave their time so generously:

Professor Hashim Ahmed, David Cahill, Dr Barbara Cleaver, Professor Prokar Dasgupta, Michelle Dixon, James & Nicola Forrester, Dr Mike Gill, Leyla Hawkins, Dr Caddy Kroll, Professor David Mabey, Dr George Peck, Sarah Jane Marsh, Dr Peter Bennie, Red Threads, Nicholas Timmins, Ron Singer, Paul Atkinson, Mick Duncan, Allyson Pollock, Bex Cowell, Alan Duddy, Everyone at the Stratford Activists' Forum, Isaac Madge, Lee Beech, Katharina Lochmann, Timothy Reichardt, Emily Fuller, Church of the Holy Spirit.

Everyone at Lakin McCarthy: Mike, Warren, Debra, Kate, Sharron, Catherine, Jamie

As always Jenny, Charlie, Izzy and Ralph.

Introduction

Hello, if you are reading this you have probably come to the show…or had a friend who came and got you the play script…or you are in a bookshop with a theatre section…or a charity shop with no central vetting for books…or you have stolen it…anyway, anyway it doesn't matter even if you stole the book… Welcome and I hope you enjoy it.

In making this show I'd talk to anyone and everyone who would have me, and each evening I would come home and regale my family with the stories and conversations I had just witnessed. To retell all the stories would take a stage show that lasted two days, I do not have the skill and you do not have the patience to do that. And as yet no theatre has had the inclination either, leaving a heap of discarded tales that have influenced the show but never get to bask in the spotlight of the telling of them.

Then I was asked to write an introduction…

One of the things that really struck me making this show was how much people were prepared to give up their time for this institution. Whether it was the group of people fighting the government's new plans for ACOs and STPs through the courts or the radiologist who overheard me talking to a friend on the tube and said, 'I might be able to shed some light on your discussion,' she then made contact through my website and later phoned me to talk me through the crisis in staffing for radiologists (part of which is an increased work load and no increase in staffing levels).

I attended one meeting of activists in a community centre in Stratford. It was an incredible hour and a half, listening to junior doctors, consultants, GPs and patients talk about the stresses they faced in and with the NHS. One paediatrician spoke of a situation where parents with sharp elbows found it easier to navigate the NHS and the inverse law of health meant that those who needed it most would be the ones who found it hardest to get the help they needed. The room was brought to tears by a young oncologist movingly explaining how privatised cleaning staff would barge into the room when she was delivering bad news and how angry that robbing of dignity made her. Not with the cleaners. They were just doing their job under the terms they've been given. Someone else spoke of the under staffing and the strain it was putting on everyone – we are 40,000 nurses understaffed in the NHS and 10,000 doctors short too. The last person to speak, as the clock ticked on and community centre staff began to mutter about stacking chairs, a man who had been silent all evening said, 'I take the fact we have not mentioned mental health as indicative of its low priority in the NHS.'

We had barely time to register what he said before it was time to leave.

After the meeting had finished and we had left the building I chatted to this man, a psychologist, by a duel carriage way in Stratford catching the evening sun and the nitrous oxide. He is so outraged that the NHS is failing so many mental health patients that rather than just moan about it he has abandoned his own practice. He now runs free therapy for the unemployed and low waged. He does not limit the number of sessions to the usual eight sessions of CBT (Cognitive Behavioural Therapy) as the NHS does but has open ended treatment. People can come for as long as they need to. He runs this free service out of community centres and at one stage a shopping mall. He organises other psychologists to give up their time to follow suit, most cannot give up their practice entirely but they can offer one or two sessions a week and a small community organisation is beginning to build up.

I asked him what it was that inspired this and he said, 'The Occupy movement.'

I just wanted to take this moment to point to this story that for reasons of time will not make it into the show. A man so frustrated by the state of mental health provision in this country that he treats people for free in shopping centres.

The NHS is a magnificent entity that is in crisis and is held together by the incredible good will of the staff, now more than ever it needs proper funding levels, proper staffing levels and critical friends.

Salut and thanks to all those in the NHS who allowed me to witness their professionalism and kindness.

Mark Thomas

Preface

This show has been two years in the making. It came about through a chance meeting in 2016 when Mark Thomas came to see *Drones, Baby, Drones* which I had directed at the Arcola, and casually said we should work together and did I have any ideas? I jumped at the chance and told him that I was very interested in doing something about the NHS for its 70th anniversary – little suspecting this anniversary would become a huge national event.

In Spring 2017 we approached the Wellcome Trust and they generously agreed to fund the research for the show. Thus began a long journey talking to scores of people working, day to day, with patients in the NHS and academics, scientists and policy advisers concerned with the nation's health. We owe a huge debt in the making of this play to the eight public figures who also kindly agreed to be interviewed for the play in theatres around the country; as well as to the staff of the Imperial College Healthcare NHS Trust (St Mary's, Charing Cross and Hammersmith Hospitals) who were so welcoming and generous with their time during Mark's residency there.

Most particularly we are grateful to Dr Barbara Cleaver who inspired us and opened so many doors for us at the outset of the project, and to Michelle Dixon whose enthusiasm and dedication to the NHS made the Imperial College residency so effective.

My own journey during the making this play has been somewhat ambivalent. By chance for much of the early period of our research I was a patient at UCLH, St Mary's and Charing Cross hospitals and perhaps saw the workings of the NHS at rather closer proximity than I would have wished. The care and understanding with which I was treated would have been revelatory and amazing had not my past encounters with the NHS been similarly caring and extraordinary.

We are roughly the same age, we have grown up together, and I always taken it for granted that the state will look after me in ill health, and for the most part it has done that brilliantly. There have been the odd blips and bureaucratic confusions, but in an organisation that is the fifth largest employer in the world that is inevitable. However I am on the more affluent end of a graph on health differentials and it is at the other end where the largest disparity of health outcomes has been most clearly evidenced and should most urgently be addressed. The figures mentioned in this play speak for themselves.

Our research for the play has clearly revealed a number of common themes, but perhaps paramount among them are three:

1. If we value our nation's and our own health we need to pay much more for it through taxation.

2. We need to ensure that the NHS gets a proper settlement over ten years without more politically inspired changes and reforms.

3. We need to fund the social care budget adequately so that the elderly and those with physical and mental difficulties have proper care without worry or fear.

During these eighteen months of research, sometimes as a patient but mainly for the play, I have come to the conclusion that we have a right, indeed a duty, to be critical of a properly funded NHS, but with the lack of resources under which the NHS has struggled this winter it is a minor miracle that the service has coped so well, and it is entirely due to the devotion and dedication of so many of its staff. They work under huge pressure, with great care and often selflessly, may we all cherish them more and treat them better – this play is dedicated to their work.

Nicolas Kent
Co-Producer & Director

Creative Team

PERFORMER, WRITER &
CO-PRODUCER, Mark Thomas

DIRECTOR & CO-PRODUCER, Nicolas Kent

CO-PRODUCER & TOUR MANAGEMENT,
Lakin McCarthy

SET, VIDEO & LIGHTING DESIGN, Jon Driscoll

SOUND DESIGN, Helen Atkinson

RESEARCHER, Susan McNicholas

REHEARSAL STAGE &
PRODUCTION MANAGER, Miki Jablkowska

TOUR PRODUCTION MANAGER, Tine Selby

INTERVIEW FILMING, Thea Stevenson

GRAPHIC DESIGN, Greg Matthews

WEB CONSTRUCTION, Jack Gamble

INTERVIEW PUBLICIST, Veronica Pasteur

PUBLICIST, Bex Cowell

Writer and Performer   MARK THOMAS

MARK THOMAS has earnt his living as a performer for thirty-three years.

Director   NICOLAS KENT

NICOLAS KENT graduated from St Catharine's College, Cambridge in 1967 with an English degree. He started his career at Liverpool Playhouse in 1967 as an ABC TV trainee regional theatre director. In 1970 he became Artistic Director of the Watermill Theatre, from 1970-72 Associate Director of the Traverse Theatre, Edinburgh and from 1976-81 Administrative Director of The Oxford Playhouse Company. From 1984-2012 he was Artistic Director of the Tricycle Theatre in London.

He has directed productions in over 100 theatres around the world including the West End and New York; as well as for notable companies in Great Britain including the National Theatre, The Royal Shakespeare Company, the Royal Court, the Donmar Warehouse, the Hampstead Theatre, the Lyric Theatre Hammersmith and the Young Vic.

He is probably best known for the political work he did at Tricycle Theatre, where the verbatim plays he directed became known as the Tricycle Tribunal plays, and included *The Colour of Justice (the Stephen Lawrence Inquiry)*, *Nuremberg*, *Srebrenica*, *Bloody Sunday* (Olivier Award for

Special Achievement), *Guantanamo* & *The Riots*. Most of which were broadcast by the BBC, and two which were performed in the Houses of Parliament and on Capitol Hill. In 2009 directed the nine-hour trilogy *The Great Game – Afghanistan* which was nominated for an Olivier award in London, and subsequently toured the USA; as well as two command performances for the Pentagon in Washington in 2011. One year later he directed a two part eight play series looking at the history of nuclear deterrence: *The Bomb: a partial history*.

He has also directed many plays in the USA: both regionally and in New York. He has directed and produced many plays for the BBC and Channel 4 television. In the Autumn of 2015 his seven-play series *The Price of Oil* was broadcast for BBC Radio 4.

In 2016 he directed *Another World* at the National Theatre and *Drones, Baby, Drone*s at the Arcola Theatre.

In 2017 he edited & directed his own play *All the President's Men?* in a co-production between the Public Theater in New York & the National Theatre in London for a special staged reading in the West End and on Broadway with Alec Baldwin & Ellen Burstyn.

He has an honorary doctorate from Westminster University, was the first person to be awarded the Freedom of the London Borough of Brent, and whilst at the Tricycle

Theatre won an Evening Standard special award for Pioneering Political Theatre as well as the 2011 Liberty Human Rights Arts Award.

Producers   LAKIN MCCARTHY

MIKE MCCARTHY and WARREN LAKIN have a combined experience of more than sixty years as performers, directors and producers in the fields of touring theatre, comedy and music.

Designer   JON DRISCOLL

JON DRISCOLL studied Cinematography at the National Film and Television School, Beaconsfield and Theatre Design at Croydon College of Art.

His designs for theatre include; *3 Winters, King Lear, The Effect, People, The Last of the Haussmans, Travelling Light, Earthquakes in London, Nation, The Power of Yes, All's Well That Ends Well, The Observer, Gethsemane, Her Naked Skin, Fram, A Matter of Life and Death* and *The Reporter* for the National. *INK, Little Eyolf, The Lightning Play* and *Whistling Psyche* for the Almeida. *Brief Encounter* for Kneehigh (Obie Award, LA Drama Critics Circle Award and Olivier nomination). *Mack and Mabel, ENRON* (Olivier nomination), *Separate Tables* and *The Last Cigarette* for Chichester. *The Winter's Tale* and *Harlequinade* for the Kenneth Branagh Company. *Richard III, The Prisoner of*

Second Avenue and *Complicit* for the Old Vic and *Frost/ Nixon* for the Donmar.

West End designs include *Charlie and the Chocolate Factory* (Olivier Award), *Ghost the Musical* (also Broadway; Drama Desk Award and Tony Nomination), *The Exorcist, Stephen Ward, From Here to Eternity, The King's Speech, The Wizard of Oz, Love Never Dies, Dirty Dancing, Our House, Up for Grabs* and *Dance of Death*.

Broadway designs include *Finding Neverland* and *Chaplin the Musical* (Drama Desk nomination). *Sousatzka* Toronto. Dance designs include *Alice's Adventures in Wonderland* for the Royal Ballet (Olivier nomination).

Opera designs include *Carmen* at the Santa Fe Opera.

Concert and Events designs include *The Phantom of the Opera* at the Royal Albert Hall, Secret Cinema's *Blade Runner* and Kate Bush's Before the Dawn at the Hammersmith Apollo.

Sound Designer   HELEN ATKINSON

HELEN ATKINSON's sound designs for Mark Thomas include: *Bravo Figaro & Cuckooed*.

Other recent designs include: *Grief is a thing with Feathers* (Complicite) *2nd Violinist* (Landmark & Wide Open Opera); *Salomé* (RSC); *Arlington* (Landmark and Galway International Arts Festival); *The Suicide* (Lyttleton, National

Theatre); *Much Ado about Nothing* (Queens Theatre, Hornchurch); *You for Me for You* (Royal Court Upstairs); *The Last Hotel* (Landmark and Wide Open Opera); *The Matchbox* (Galway International Arts Festival); *Ballyturk,* for which she was awarded Best Sound Designer at the 2014 Irish Times Irish Theatre Awards (Landmark and Galway International Arts Festival); *The Edge, 1001 Nights, As You Like It* and *Elegy* (Transport); *The Summerbook,* *'Twas the Night before Christmas* and *1001 nights* (Unicorn Theatre); *Deep Blue Sea*, *All My Sons* and *Of Mice and Men* (Watermill Theatre); *Mr Whatnot* and *A Christmas Carol* (Northampton Theatre Royal); *Macbeth* (Cheek by Jowl); *Mountaineering* and *You'll See Me Sailing in Antarctica* (Non Zero One); *Wolfschild, Great Night Out* and *Once Upon a Castle (Wildworks); Peppa Pig's Surprise* and *Octonauts and the Deep Sea Volcano Adventure* (Firey Light).

Rehearsal Production Manager   MIKI JABLOWSKA

MIKI JABLOWSKA has worked principally in automation on West End musicals such as *Miss Saigon, Ghost, Jersey Boys, Spamalot, Les Misérables* (Paris).

Tour Production Manager   TINE SELBY

TINE SELBY has spent the first thirty-one years of her career mucking about in various aspects of the arts and entertainment industry, including theatre-in-education, venue-based technical and operational work and music and arts festivals, both in the UK and abroad.

Currently she is tour production manager for Mark Thomas and Ruby Wax, and not at home very much.

In Pictures

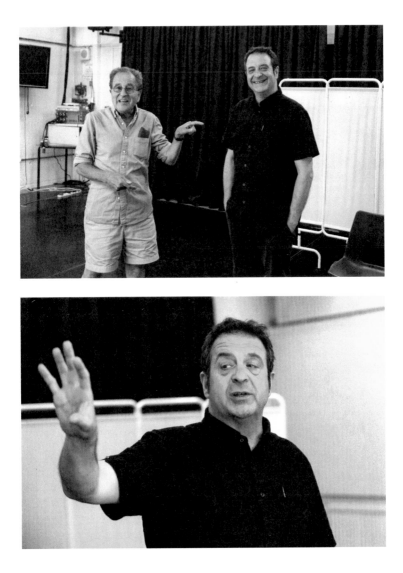

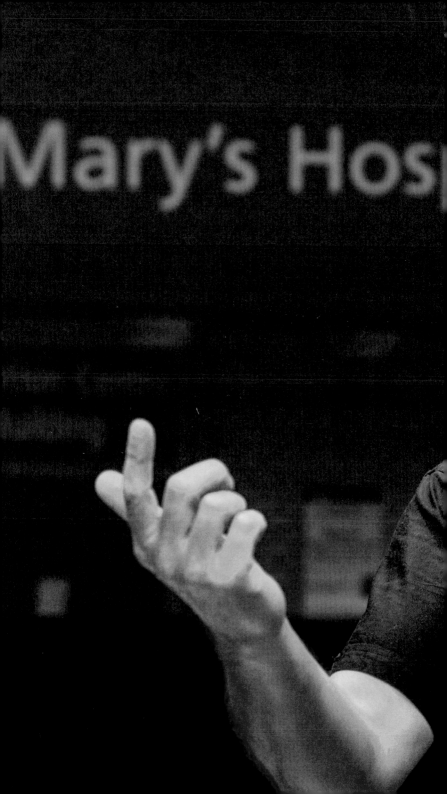

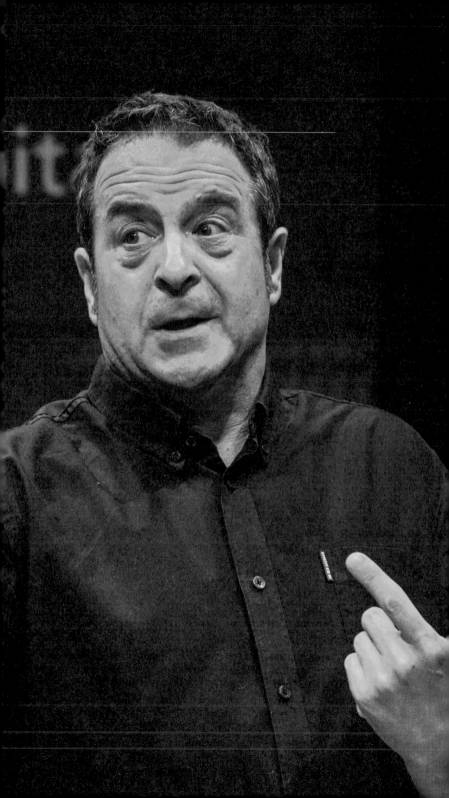

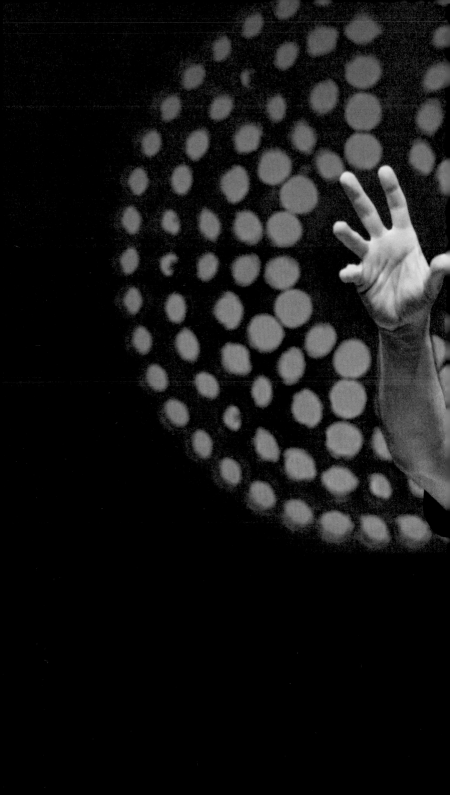

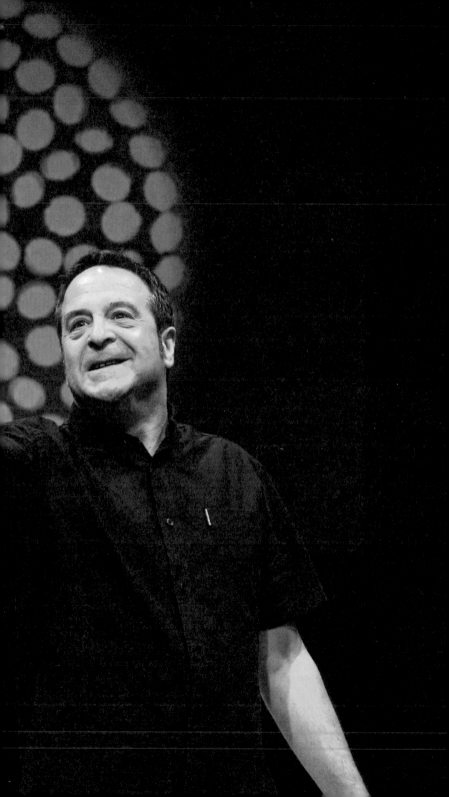

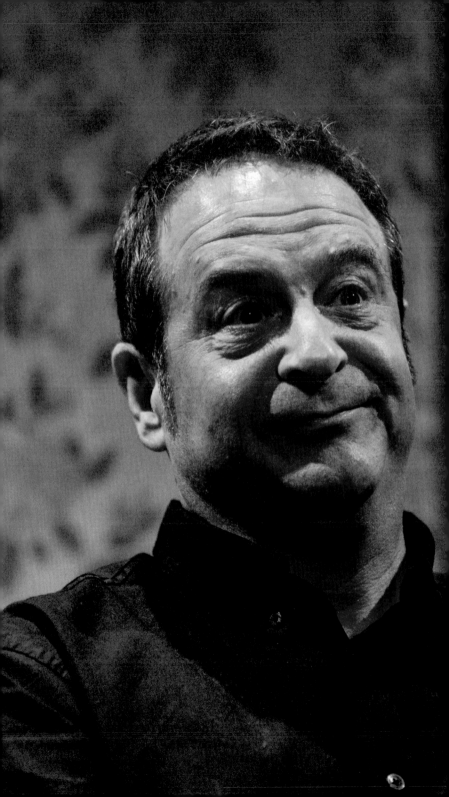

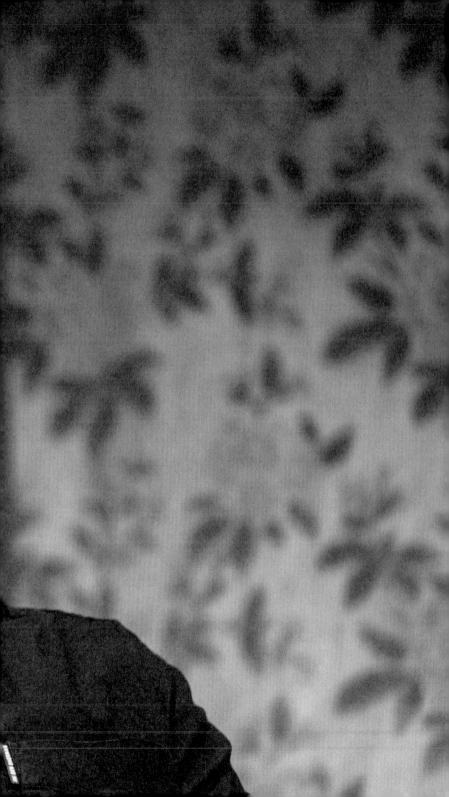

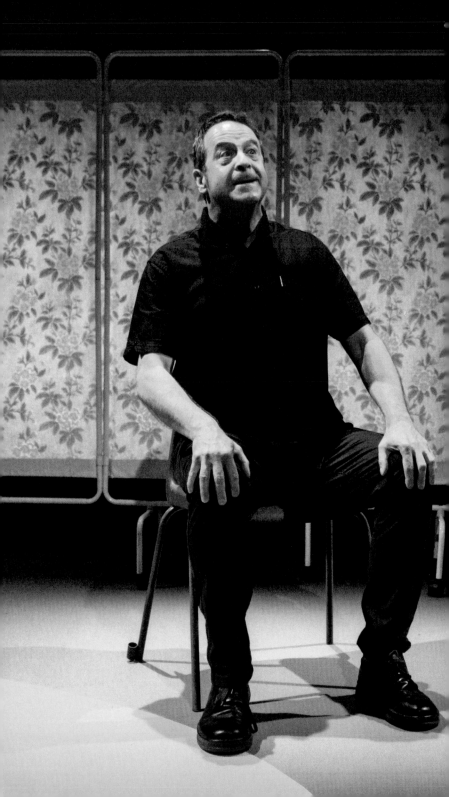

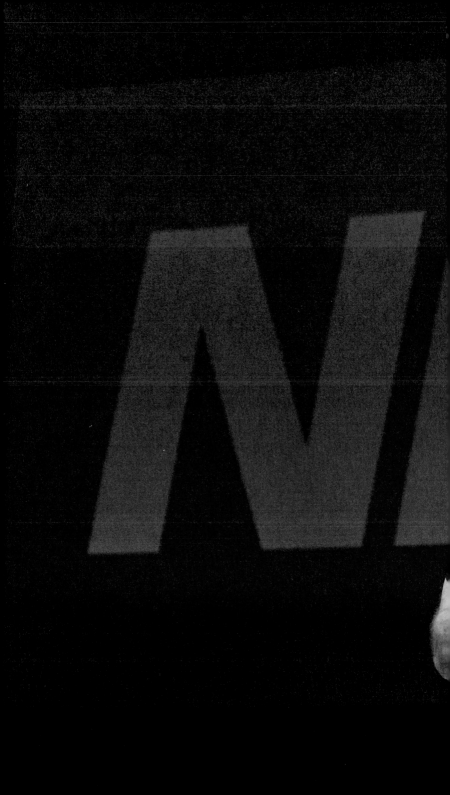

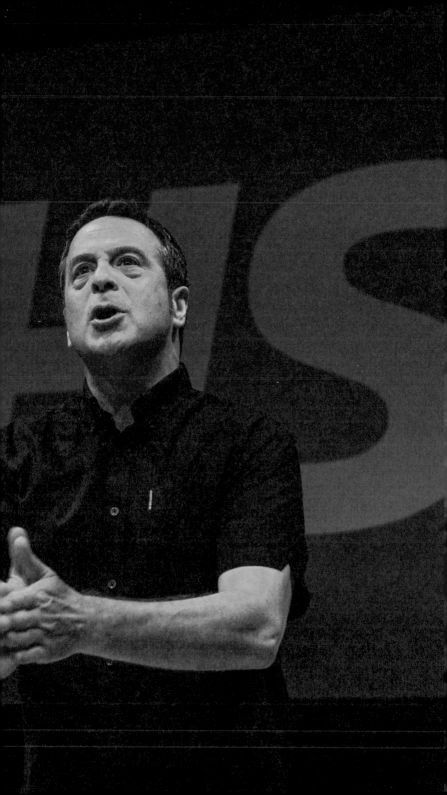

Onstage a four-panel hospital screen stage left and a plastic chair in front of it. Downstage right a hospital trolley on wheels. A projection screen at the back of the stage.

Footage of the entrance to Lisson Grove Health Centre, with a caption saying 'The view from the rehearsal room,' is played on a screen whilst audience are seated.

Screen changes and Pathé fanfare & newsreel plays:

'A HEALTHIER BRITAIN

It's coming.

It's on the way.

Look out for it'

V/O: This leaflet is coming through your letterbox one day soon or maybe you've already had your copy. Read it carefully. It tells you what the new National Health Service is.'

Lights go down and intro fanfare replays. Lights go up and MARK enters.

My mum remembers seeing that, she remembers the creation of the NHS, she says,

'Your nan was thrilled.'

My grandmother came from North Seaton, the North East, from a mining family. All her stories were about bullies and physical calamity.

She told me how they lived in a row of miners' houses owned by the mining company and she remembered when the company installed electricity, so the miners' families had electric lights for the first time but the company didn't give them any switches. The company kept the switch. And 4.30pm in the winter they switch on the lights in every house, 9.30pm time for bed and all the lights go out.

She told me that when there was an accident at pit an alarm was sounded and the families would stand in the street by their front doors, and the medical cart would come down the street bearing the injured and/or dead, about how they were terrified that the cart would stop at their door, because then it was your relatives in there. And she said how she felt enormous relief when it passed mixed with intense guilt that she had wished misfortune on the people further down the street.

Her family used to save a penny a week in a cup on the shelf for the doctor and if a child was ill there was a discussion about whether they should call the doctor and spend the money or save it until someone else was worse.

The NHS was founded in 1948 on three principles, it should be free, comprehensive – everything is covered – and universal – for everyone.

Health Minister Nye Bevan, the father of the NHS, said the NHS was created, 'In Place of Fear.'

'In Place of Fear.'

And in its first two years of existence between 1948 and 1950 it prescribed – well guess how many pairs of glasses the NHS prescribed for free in its first two years?

Seventeen million pairs of glasses.

Seventeen million people who could read and see properly. And my grandmother was one of them.

For seventy years the NHS has not just fought illness but *fear*.

Like 45,000,000 others I was born under the NHS. I was born in St Thomas's hospital on the south bank of the Thames opposite Parliament. I was literally born screaming at politicians. And here I am today…

I was born to a nurse, my mum was a midwife, she trained in Glasgow in the Gorbals in 1957. She told me stories of delivering babies in tenements and there was no crib or cot so she would wrap the baby in swaddling and put it in drawer. Health and wealth have always been entwined.

Everyone says the NHS needs more money, you can't turn on *Question Time* without someone declaring they would be happy to pay a 1p in the pound tax increase IF the money was ring-fenced for the NHS – by the end of the show I hope to prove that argument wrong.

Everyone says it needs more money, even our Prime Minister agrees and is increasing funding to the NHS as a birthday present, a present! Only the Tories can spend our tax money and call it a present.

Everyone I spoke to in the NHS said this money is not enough and will barely get the service back to where it was ten years ago, let alone improve it.

Nearly everyone I spoke to talked of how this year, the celebratory year, has been the most difficult, people working in mental health spoke of the service buckling under the pressure and they point to the fact only four in ten people with a mental illness get any kind of treatment on the NHS. Four in ten. If that was cancer there would be uproar ... And for two weeks this year the NHS was in special measures.

My family worked in the NHS. I was born in the NHS and it is very possible that I will die in the NHS and I want to know what state it is going to be in when I need it most.

To do this I do three things:

I conduct a series of public interviews with academics and practitioners to see where the NHS is now and where it could be.

I spend a month in residency at the Imperial College Healthcare Trust which has four NHS hospitals in West London, shadowing consultants, doctors and nurses.

And finally I talk to a doctor to assess what could go wrong for me over the coming years. What will drive me into the arms of the NHS.

The results are this show,

CHECK-UP: Our NHS @ 70.

***

Doctor Ron is a retired GP from Tower Hamlets in London and I spend an afternoon with him to ask what could go wrong with me.

MARK (AS RON): *'Everything. Anything. You're fifty-five now Mark. The only things you don't* *have to worry about are milk teeth and the*

menopause. Other than that everything is coming

at you. Now when you die you want to go quick.

You don't want to linger, don't hang about, you

don't want to end up in hospital, nasty places,

people die there. An accident. Run over by a car.

Nice and quick. A bus would be more certain.

Or a mirror on the side of the bus. Back of the

head. Bang. Wouldn't even see it coming. Out.

You're a cyclist. And I bet you don't stop at red

lights. Boom! Travis Perkins scaffold lorry. Over.'

   MARK walks to trolley, gets soap from dispenser
   attached to trolley and cleans hands.

Armed with that cheery thought I head for

my second day at St Mary's, Paddington. I am

scheduled to be there from 5pm to 6.30pm

to tour Major Trauma. There are four major

trauma centres in London, if you get shot

stabbed, have serious head injuries, are in a car crash or involved in a terrorist attack, one of these is where you go. The man I am shadowing is Dr Asif Rahman, he is from Fife and to any Scots in the audience I apologise in advance for the accent.

MARK (AS RAHMAN): *'Right, you need to understand the colour of the scrubs. Senior consultants wear purple scrubs. This is Jane, she's in purple, senior consultant for A & E tonight, Jane is ex- army. We like ex-army. So Senior Consultant – purple, doctors – green, nurses – blue, senior nurses – dark blue and just for clarity some doctors – blue. I'm in charge of Resus tonight.'*

Resus is an extension to A&E. The area is quite small, six bays, three each side, divided by concertinaed paper curtains. At one end is a nurses' station with some computers and a TV screen with a live CCTV feed onto the ambulance bay.

MARK (AS RAHMAN): *'When a patient comes in my job is to organise the team, assign a doctor who leads the team, what people we need, what equipment and call on the expertise of surgeons and consultants in the hospital who we might need.'*

'It seems pretty quiet…'

'Do not use the 'Q' word. You used the 'Q' word!'

The alarm goes. Ambulance drivers bring in a man strapped to a gurney loudly chanting, *'1.2.3.1.2.3.1.2.3.1.2.3.'*

'Appears to be a coping strategy.'

Dr Rahman in purple stands at the end of the bed, a doctor in blue beside him. Ambulance do the handover,

'Fifty-one year old male, epileptic seizure, fallen down some stairs, head injury and suspected broken shoulder. Alcohol issues, traces of diazepam around his mouth and PTSD. '

'1.2.3. 1.2.3. 1.2.3.'

'Okay do you know what happened?'

'Epilepsy and diazepam.'

'Is there anything else wrong?'

'Yes'

'Can you tell me?'

'Can't remember. 1.2.3. 1.2.3. 1.2.3.'

'PLAN!'

The word PLAN is clearly shouted each time there's new instructions for treatment as the patient's circumstances change.

This plan is an MRI on the head and shoulder.

On my first day a nurse told me, *'If you end up in a hot spot make sure you are well hydrated and have eaten a banana, because if you faint, that is a trip hazard.'*

Two alarms go off. Dr Rahman sorts out stretcher, pushes the equipment in the bay and starts to organise teams.

'Two are coming in. One I'm not too worried about, fractured skull but steady heart beat. The other one I am worried about a head injury and dropping heart rate.'

An elderly woman is wheeled in, head in bandages and blood everywhere. And I am extremely glad I have had a banana.

A team head to the CCTV.

The second patient arrives and I try and take up as little room as possible. Police are gathered in one corner. The air ambulance doctor in orange stands next to the purple scrubs of Dr Rahman.

'HANDOVER.'

'Forty-year-old woman, gone through first floor window, landed concrete patio, head injuries, internal bleeding and there is lots of glass around her clothing – be careful.'

'DOUBLE GLOVING, EVERYONE. DOUBLE GLOVING.'

'PLAN.'

'Tube her, blood and plasma. Heart rate going down. Porter more blood please and quickly.'

Surgeons from other departments arrive to see if they will be needed. I stand opposite the bay next to a WPC, the police officer is my colour chart, if her face is looking less than rose then so am I.

'She's dropping, CPR now please.'

A nurse in dark blue rhythmically pumps the woman's heart. The air ambulance have gone. Other surgeons arrive. Suddenly *'1.2.3., 1.2.3., 1.2.3.'* comes from the next bay inches way.

'Help me, help me!'

'PLAN.'

'She's bleeding internally. Let's drain this. Laparotomy, each side.'

A laparotomy is a cut made into the side of the abdomen to drain internal bleed and find its source. One cut left and right. Blood splashes on the floor. The cop is white and so am I.

'Tube please.'

A tube is attached to the woman's side and a plastic container fills up with blood.

'PLAN.'

My plan is to get as far away as possible and get a glass of water.

'PLAN.'

'Moving to surgery. Now please. Mark follow me.'

Suddenly I am running behind a bed and doctors, nurses, tubes and blood through the corridor. We get to the lift. A lift door opens and it's full of visitors holding gifts of bears and flowers.

'EVERYONE OUT NOW PLEASE!'

There isn't enough room for everyone so the WPC, a doctor and me run up the stairs into theatre. Dr Rahman turns to the WPC,

'Wait outside, please. Mark, you can stand in the corner.'

BRIGHT LIGHTS COME UP ON THE OPERATING TABLE.

On the operating table the woman is laid out cruciform, covered in green sheets, large circular lights above her. Doctors and nurses work around her. Dr Rahman in purple writes the notes for the team and surgeons take over.

'Could someone open the door so the doctors in scrubs can hear?'

Next to me is a pressure pad. I look up. Dr Asif Rahman nods, I press the pad and the door opens so the doctors in scrubs can hear the plan and I am hugely relieved I have done a tiny action to help and am no longer entirely a bystander.

There must be twenty people in the room, surgeons with magnifying optics trying to find the source of the bleeding, doctors draining fluids, anaethetists, nurses preparing bandages, sutures, needles, medical equipment, a nurse doing a blood transfusion with a surgical matt on the floor onto which he places empty blood bags so they know how much blood is going in. Including the air ambulance, paramedics, police and hospital staff there must be thirty-five people trying to save her life.

And she dies.

The two stabbings who came in, the two cyclists versus cars, the old woman with a fractured skull and Mr *'1.2.3.'* live.

It is 9.30pm and I am waiting in a corridor. I have left my bag and coat in Dr Asif Rahman's room. He is in another room telling the woman's family what has happened.

He appears and says, *'Let's get your bag and coat,'* and we start to head up the stairs to his office.

I mutter something about never have seen such a Herculean effort…

He says, *'I blame you for you this, you used the Q word.'*

I have a severe sense of humour failure and I think my lower lip wobbles.

'I'm just joking, I'm just joking.'

And I get my coat and my bag. I get the tube. I go home, I get changed. I go to sleep and am woken in the morning by my son shouting,

'Who's eaten all the bananas?!'

The amazing thing about A&E is that it is classless. It does not matter who you are – if you come in through that door you will get the best possible treatment they can offer.

Except class has a way of sorting people out before anyone has even walked through the A&E door.

***

The first public interview I did was with Professor Michael Marmot, author of a ground-breaking report on health inequalities, on why some people live longer than others. In the photo there is a guitar next to him because we interviewed him on the set of a pantomime. I now believe all interviews should take place on panto sets. I want to see Boris stepping out of a pumpkin carriage… and onto a scaffold… And that's why Amnesty won't let me join.

MARK sits on plastic chair, photograph of Professor Sir Michael Marmot is projected onto the hospital screen stage right and on the large screen the words 'Professor Sir Michael Marmot' in very large letters over the top.

As a government expert and academic I expect him to be dry and crispy but actually he's not. He's furious.

MARK (AS MARMOT): '*Most of the determinants of health lie outside of the NHS. The things that affect health outcomes are housing, poor housing effects health, education, a child's first eight years we know are crucial to health outcomes, unemployment, anxiety through job insecurity, poor diet. All these things affect health outcomes. The poorer you are the more likely you are to suffer from ill health. And those determinants start at birth and stay with you throughout your life unless we intervene. We condemn people to an early death and poor health.*

When my report was launched, in central London, Gordon Brown used the example that

*if you got on the central line at Holborn and
headed East life expectancy goes down by one year
for every stop. The London tube map is a map
of health differentials. But I'll give you a current
example. Grenfell.'*

The facts are that people who live in the area
near Grenfell and those who live the streets
around Harrods – the same London Borough,
the difference in life expectancy between
Grenfell and Harrods…is twenty-two years.
People in the poor areas around Grenfell die
twenty-two years earlier.

*'And I look upon this as a moral issue not an
economic one. If you judge, <u>and I do judge</u>,
that we can avoid these health outcomes with
reasonable measures and we do not avoid them
that is unjust. People are being robbed of years of
life and quality of life.'*

MARK walks to trolley, gets soap from dispenser attached to trolley and cleans hands.

Our first encounter for health issues is normally with a GP and the new NHS structure created by the 2012 Lansley Act puts them as gatekeepers to the rest of the NHS. Except one million people a week have problems getting an appointment with a GP. The average wait is thirteen days. Not so Dr Jackie Applebee. She is a GP in Tower Hamlets, one of the poorest parts of London. Her patients do not wait thirteen days for an appointment because she has a daily walk-in surgery.

The name 'Dr Jackie Applebee' is projected onto the large screen.

MARK (AS JACKIE): *'People know they might have to wait an hour or an hour and a half but if they turn up they will be seen.'*

I ask,

'Are there any qualifiers, a criterion for the walk-in service?'

'Yes… People feel they need to see a doctor.'

She lives and breathes the service, when she makes a cup of tea she tells me,

'What gets me is with the cuts and underfunding… I know this sounds small but they have cut the toe nail cutting service for older people. If they can't bend over someone needs to cut their toenails and now it's gone. And what it is that upsets me most is that it is just mean… do you want milk?'

The consulting room feels familiar. Family picture, red rubbish bin, yellow sharps bin, a corporate calendar, a notice about 'Diabetes and Ramadan' and a pile of leaflets on the desk for the 'Save the NHS' demo.

Now I know this should be a captive audience but I can't see how she is going to hand out many of these. *'The test results read all clear. Would you like to go on a march?'*

Over two days, she sees twenty-one patients who agree for me to be present, she does telephone conference calls with specialists and teams, does six phone calls to patients, prescribes three sets of antibiotics, refuses a repeat prescription for codeine, twice hands out tissues when patients weep when revealing their situation and covers everything from earache to duodenal ulcers. I am amazed at the level of concentrated decision-making. She says,

'The art is to make sure you treat the last patient in as if they were the first one in that morning.'

A young man comes in, he has perfect timing.

'How can I help you?'

'I've got a dry cough. Had it for two weeks. Won't go away.*cough cough*'

'Okay...let's have a look. Breathe in. Breathe out...It looks like it is viral and should clear up but if it goes on for another two weeks come back. Had any other illness recently?'

'Viral meningitis in November. I was in America.'

'America?'

'San Francisco. I spent six days in hospital.'

Goodness and so you had a lumbar puncture?'

'I had fifteen.'

'Fifteen lumbar punctures!?!'

'Fifteen. They couldn't get it right. In the end they gave me a patient advocate to deal with the doctors and the insurance.'

'Well we don't want that happening over here.'

And she hands him a leaflet!

***

A caption is projected on the large screen & a photograph on the small screen: Professor Dame Sally Davies, Chief Medical Officer for England.

Public Health is the domain of the Chief Medical Officer and England's CMO is Professor Dame Sally Davies, the first female Chief Medical Officer. Her job is to spot health threats to the general population and advise government on how to stop them. I like her partly because the *Daily Mail* had a pop at her and anyone the *Daily Mail* has had a pop at surely has some good points. She issued advice on safe levels of units of alcohol and the *Daily Mail* started bleating 'nanny state'. Chatting to her she comes over a bit like Clare Balding – but not snide. She has published reports on air pollution and child mental health and social media but what is really exercising her at the moment is…

'… Antimicrobial resistance. Bacteria is doing what it does – evolve defences against the things that attack it… antibiotics.

700,000 people die each year globally because the drugs aren't working anymore.

We use antibiotics to treat infection in everything from a cut finger to minor surgery and beyond, so if antibiotics fail medical science goes back a century. And if we carry on as we are, it's estimated that 700,000 figure will jump to ten million. In thirty years. That's bigger than cancer.

Sally points to the culprits – some of it is over-prescription especially globally but mainly it's the food industry. It's cheaper than hygiene. 80% of America's antibiotic use is in farming.

'*When I was working with the World Health Organisation panel on anti-microbial resistance, samples from the river Ganges were tested and they found concentrations of antibiotics higher than you would expect to find in a human*

bloodstream from someone on a course of
antibiotics.'

During questions someone from the audience
asks…

   SFX: Recording of audience member: 'If I buy
   organic milk will there be antibiotics in it?'

'There shouldn't be, if you buy organic
milk or meat it should be free of chemicals.
Prince Charles treats his herd of cattle
homoeopathically…'

'Homeopathic cows! Princes Charles has
homeopathic cows. Was this in the news? Does he
have chickens do they get acupuncture? How do
you know about his homeopathic cows?'

There is an awkward silence then the CMO
says…

'I've meet them and very healthy they seem too.'

We could and should develop new drugs – there's been no new antibiotics since the 1980s but there is no incentive for big Pharma to do that – there's no money in developing an antibiotic as a last line of resistance. No one bothers.

When I ask her about how you take on industry and force change she says, '*it's about socialising the argument*'. Who am I to argue with the CMO but surely when you're dealing with pharma and industries like alcohol, oil and sugar I don't want to socialise an argument, I want industry regulated out of the 19th century.

Alcohol – over a million alcohol related admissions in NHS England a year.

Air pollution – 40,000 deaths annually in UK from air pollution.

Sugar – second fattest people in Europe after Hungary (home of the dumpling), two thirds of adults and one in four kids overweight. Obesity costs the NHS £6.1bn a year, societally including unemployment benefits etc it costs us £27bn a year. By the time the NHS is 100 the figure is set to rise to £50bn, half the current NHS budget.

In thirty years time we will look back at repeats of *The Great British Bake Off* and think, how the fuck did they get away with that? It's *Trainspotting* for Middle England. Sugar kills more than cooking heroin and snorting coke. One of the companies is called *Silver Spoon!* How much more obvious does it have to be?!

MARK (AS RON): *'You're fat. Two stone overweight. Say a stone and a half with a good fitting shirt. You are possibly pre-diabetic. You might lose weight. You'll probably put it back it again. Bang - Diabetes. On medication for the rest of your life. Increased risk of heart attack, stroke. Cancer. Then come the amputations. A couple of toes. A foot. It could go all the way to the knee.'*

MARK walks to the trolley and cleans his hands.

In the Surgical Innovation Centre at St Mary's Hospital.

Points to screen where there is a caption:

Mr Ahmed Ahmed (Consultant Surgeon specialising in Laparoscopic, Gastrointestinal and Bariatric surgery, Charing Cross and St Mary's Hospitals.

This is Mr Ahmed Ahmed, so good they named him twice.

MARK (AS AHMED): *'Okay, Mark, let's get you in scrubs and find yourself a pair of crocs in the changing room.'*

Crocs! Doctors and cooks are the only people who can wear Crocs. Civilians never. Crocs as leisure wear is a public declaration of failure, it says I have no ambition nor sex life and I don't care who knows.

The changing room has a delicate whiff of body odour. Which is vaguely comforting as it reminds me of dressing rooms. It is also deeply disturbing to discover Crocs are comfortable.

MARK (AS AHMED): *'I am going to perform keyhole surgery today. It's called a gastric sleeve. We enter through four incisions in the abdomen,* *then cut and staple the stomach. We will remove about 70% of the patient's stomach to create a banana shaped stomach.*

And, if there is one thing you must tell people, is obesity is not a lifestyle choice. No one chooses to be like this.

I am going to introduce you to the patient I am operating on. He has agreed to see you. He is thirty-five, 178 kilos which is 28 stone. Can't work, can barely walk, has diabetes and depression. After the surgery we expect to see 20%-30% weight loss, not slim but he can go back to work, he will be productive. Hopefully beat the cycle of depression and come off the diabetes medicines. It will change his life.'

I ask the man what he hopes for after the procedure:

'Well I want to go back to work, lead a normal life but most of all I've got an eleven-year-old daughter who worries everyday that I am going to die. And I just want a normal relationship with her.'

In the tea room before the operation Mr Ahmed explains:

'Some will tell you to be a surgeon you need an ego, you need to be a bit of an extrovert that performing surgery in the theatre is a performance but what you need is a good anaesthetist, a surgeon and an anaesthetist work together like a double act.'

Another doctor who will be observing today pipes up, she says:

'I'm going to be performing stand-up in two weeks' time. My friends booked me down for a

five-minute slot. I have never done it before I am terrified … must be the most difficult job in the world. I figured I would talk at people, some people think I am funny and I have two jokes but if I talk really fast then I should get through it.'

Another doctor walks in and says:

'Where is this comedy chap we have with us?'

'Hi.'

'Didn't recognise you. You scrub up well.'

Bright lights come up.

In the theatre the patient is laid out upon the table, covered in green sheets with his abdomen exposed, the anaesthetist stands at the head end, monitors around him, large screens at eye level relay the interior of the patient. From somewhere some music is playing.

SFX: Music plays: 'Doin' The 68' by Roland Kirk.

'We start with four incisions, insert the portals then a rod is used to create a cavity to work in. First we are going to remove the fat attached to the stomach. That's the yellow stuff.'

For those of you who are not hydrated or have not had a banana look away now.

Footage projected onto the screen of the procedure of cutting fat from stomach.

'My glamorous assistant is going to lay the fat alongside the stomach and I'm going to cut it away using an electronically heated cutter. If you look at the screen you will see the fat bubble a little and spit sometimes even a little whisp of smoke inside the abdomen.'

Footage finishes.

Okay you can open your eyes again.

Ahmed Ahmed says,

'Come here Mark, okay now I'm going to cut away about 70% of the stomach using a tool that both cuts and staples.

Okay follow me in.

CUT…CUT…CUT…STAPLE STAPLE CUT…STAPLE CUT…STAPLE CUT STAPLE…

CUT CUT CUT…STAPLE CUT STAPLE… CUT STAPLE…AND WE'RE DONE.'

70% of the man's stomach now lies discarded in his abdomen.

*'What we do now is look for leaks. Let's have
some liquid. We are looking for bubbles, it's like
mending a puncture on a bicycle tube. That
all looks fine. Let's drain that. Then some local
anaesthetic for pain. Remove the remnants of the
stomach…then stitch him up.'*

Ahmed Ahmed inserts a pair of rods, hooks
the discarded piece of stomach, drags it across
the interior of the abdomen and starts to pull
it through the portal. And when there is about
two inches of stomach exposed, he grips it
with his hand and pulls it out like a magician
bringing a rabbit out of a hat.

  Sound cue.

All we need now is some dancing girls.

  *Projected footage of Olympic Ceremony and the
  NHS nurses dancing.*

2012 the London Olympics opening ceremony.

900 million people watch Danny Boyle place the NHS centre stage of our cultural identity.

The Culture Secretary is Jeremy Hunt.
The Health Minister, Andrew Lansley and Parliament has just passed the biggest piece of legislation to be enacted upon the NHS since it was formed.

Lansley's act abolishes the entire existing structure of the NHS. 170 organisations are shut, over 240 new ones created, over 10,000 people made redundant.

The chief exec of NHS England says the changes are so great you can see them from space.

Picture of interview with Sir Chris Ham, CEO of the King's Fund, projected on rear screen.

I speak to Chris Ham, CEO of the King's Fund, a think tank which follows health issues and I ask him,

'What ON EARTH was Lansley's thinking behind the 2012 Act?'

'Look at the early thinking when he was in opposition they were strongly influenced by experience ten, twenty years earlier when the big utilities were privatised and opened up to marketisation and he adapted that model to the NHS.'

So the structure of the NHS England is based upon the privatised British Gas?

'Based on gas, on water, on all the privatisations that took place at that time, transformed into the biggest most important public service in the country.'

The government has set the NHS against itself, in the way they did with the railways. One part of the NHS is the commissioner, they say what procedure we need and puts the contracts for them out to tender. And the other bits of the NHS compete against each other to win the contracts.

And now Lansley opens the door to 'any willing provider', so not only does the NHS have to compete in an internal market, they have to compete in an open market with the likes of Virgin Healthcare.

I'm fairly biasied so as far as I'm concerned I can only see the cons. But there must be some pros to this so I ask him what possible benefits there are to Lansley's huge reforms and Chris Ham, Chief Executive of the King's Fund says none.

NONE. So it has to be ideology.

The cost of running this market, the process of creating the tendering and bidding process, awarding contracts and administering them, well according to Chris Ham who is erring on the side of caution, it's £2bn, maybe 3. No one knows.

'Surely if we got rid of the market we would save money?'

'We would save a lot on that which is what the Scots do because they don't have to do any of this.'

We have four different models of the NHS: England, Scotland, Wales and Northern Ireland. The Scottish NHS has no market, and with the exception of three PFI hospitals has no car parking charges and no prescription charges, but house prices are going up so be quick…just parking that there.

So the next time a politician talks about inefficiency in the NHS, tell them that the inefficiency lies in the structure they created and voted for.

Projected on rear screen: Merlyn Marsden, Site Manager of Charing Cross & Hammersmith hospitals at the time of this interview.

My very first day in residency – Charing Cross hospital. Site Manager, Merlyn Marsden, shows me around.

MARK (AS MERLYN): *Don'ts and Do's.*

Don't wear jewellery: rings, bracelets, watches.

Do wear short sleeves.

Do wash you hands.

Do keep out of the way.'

She is South African by the way – I'm not just putting on an accent in case there's any casting agents in.

'This is my A&E, if you have a stroke you come here. Strokes are time sensitive. I want you up to the MRI as quickly as possible and this lift doesn't work. The patient has to come through here into the general hospital population... Hi can I help you? Up the escalator and first right... So I need a new lift. If I can get you to the MRI and diagnosed and treated and if you are fit and

healthy, we can have you walking out of here the same day. After a stroke.'

We walk past a public work of art, a woman rock climber much larger than life climbing the wall of the stairwell.

  Rock climber installation projected on rear screen.

She stops in front of it and says, *'Opinion is divided.'*

A woman comes running past us, barefoot, followed by a nurse and doctor who coax her back.

'And I need a new door. I need to keep the patients where they should be… safe so they don't wander around. I need a pad-operated door that can take knocks from the trolleys and withstand

patients tugging and pushing and pulling because they have not read the sign properly.'

'So the door is your main priority?'

'No, my main priority is beds. Flow. I need to make sure that people are moving from the hospital in good time so I can move the next patient in. More people staying in beds means less people coming in. I have a team to find out where the beds are free! Yes I need a new door and a new lift and I need to talk to the porters to see if everyone is in and we can change the lightbulbs but most of all I need flow!'

But no matter how much flow Merlyn achieves, her hospital – like the majority of others in the UK – will still end the year in deficit.

When you get paid per procedure, flow is no longer just a matter of health but finances have become entwined and when that happens everyone needs a Merlyn.

I managed to talk to two former health ministers, a minor miracle for someone who a couple of years ago was squatting MPs' second home and putting on a comedy gig to raise money for refugees. To get two former ministers shows a distinct lack of vetting.

The deficit that three quarters of our hospitals are in is due to many factors – the spending squeeze, a reduction in the tariff hospitals are paid for each procedures along with increased demand and an increase in agency fees due to a lack of staff. And PFI of course.

I talk to Blair's first health minister, Frank Dobson to ask him what was he thinking

by agreeing to PFI. Okay you have 103
new hospitals being built – and they were
hugely needed. But PFI??? How did private
consortiums building new buildings and the
NHS renting them on fixed term contracts,
allowing companies to turn up to 70% profit
on a virtually risk free investment. Quite
how you fuck up a contract like that, I do
not know but Carillion did. They have gone
bankrupt halfway through two new hospital
builds – Liverpool and Birmingham – and
once again the taxpayer has to bail out the
failure of the private sector.

*On the projection screen a freeze frame of MARK
interviewing Frank Dobson.*

I interview Dobson in a theatre above a pub.
I have a confession to make, I like him. He's
a warm and affable chap and I think why did

you ever become a politician, cos that lot will just bully you. At the end of the interview I ask him:

'What's you biggest regret as Health Minister?'

   Video tape plays Frank Dobson interview.

'Oh without a doubt PFI.'

Let's hear that again.

'What's your biggest regret?'

   Video tape plays Frank Dobson interview.

'PFI.'

And once more for clarity.

'Your biggest regret?'

   Video tape plays Frank Dobson interview.

'PFI.'

And the reason is the NHS pays £2bn a year to service that PFI debt. So you take the PFI £2bn and the £2-3bn it costs to run the market and you have got between £4-5bn which is way over Theresa May's birthday present. If you want to do something to celebrate the NHS' seventieth birthday don't bother with a gift, just don't invite the vultures to the party.

> *Projected on to the rear screen: PROFESSOR THE LORD DARZI OF DENHAM PC KBE FRS FMEDSCI HONFRENG holding the Paul Hamlyn Chair of Surgery at Imperial College London, the Royal Marsden Hospital and the Institute of Cancer Research and Director of the Institute of Global Health Innovation at Imperial College London.*

The second health minister I interview is altogether very different. Lord Darzi has an unfortunate habit of calling patients customers but he is also Director of the Institute for Global Health Innovation at Imperial College. I want to find out what we have got coming at us by way of medical innovation. Antibiotics may be failing but there must be some good news on the horizon.

I start the interview by reading out his title:

Professor The Lord Darzi of Denham PC KBE FRS FMEDSCI HONFRENG, holder of the Paul Hamlyn Chair of Surgery. Tell me have you always been an over-achiever?

He brushes off my slight with the confidence of someone used to the House of Lords' dining room.

MARK (AS LORD DARZI): *'Let me explain, over the past one hundred years medical science has doubled life expectancy. Doubled life expectancy in one hundred years. No other industry can claim that. Can banking claim that? I don't think so.*

And 40% of that innovation has come from Britain, the MRI Scan invented in Nottingham, the CT Scan, penicillin invented in the street around the corner from where I work.

And in the future we will have genomics. All of us three or four years ago had a pill, one size fits all, now because of our genetic make-up we can see which one works for each group.

We all like personalised health where you get to see the same doctor or nurse, we're talking about personalised treatment. That's revolutionary.

*Bio markers, you may have seen a blood test
which could pick up the DNA of a tumour cell
that might be circulating in the blood, before the
tumour has even grown.*

*And robotics, now some people think robotics
is surgery performed by a robot. It's not. The
greatest tool in medicine is a surgeon's hands.
The surgeon operates the machine. But there are
spaces a hand cannot get into. A robot can get
into those places.*

*And in next five years we'll have nanobots, tiny
robots you can only see under a microscope and
on their tip have chemotherapy drugs and you
can inject them and they go into the bloodstream
and target the area.*

*Going be transformational, going to have robots
you can swallow take images and biopsies and*

then Bluetooth the image to your camera, to your phone.

What greater investment can there be than health because a healthy nation is a productive nation.

You know Gordon Brown appointed me to the House of Lords and made me Health Minister, and I was talking on the Embryology and Fertility Bill when I heard a loud bang. I turned around and the Speaker of the House of Lords had had a heart attack. I rushed to him and although it has been a while I remembered my emergency training and began to administer CPR. I called for the ushers to get the defibrillator in the most un-Parliamentary language. I turn and next to me I see a woman's frock. I look up and it is the Archbishop of York praying next to me over the Speaker. I apply the pads and bang the Speaker comes back. And I couldn't help it, I turned to the Archbishop and said 'I win' and the Archbishop says, 'We did it together.'

Slide of the NHS logo projected on the rear screen.

British exceptionalism, the notion that we are superior to everyone else because we are born on an island off the coast of France, British exceptionalism has infected nearly every aspect of national discourse.

From military interventions: We're British the foreigners can't sort it out we can.

To Brexit: we're British and foreigners are invading us.

To the NHS: we're British, we don't need foreigners, oh fuck we do and more than we thought. Can we keep some?

Okay maybe not you, because you are nice people. But every single one of us is guilty of thinking the NHS is best in the world. We invented the concept of National Health. We did it first and we are the best in the world.

We are not the best. We are average. After Canada, Japan, Germany, France, Sweden – we are always after bloody Sweden, with the exception of one football match. You put an average amount of money in and we get an average set of health outcomes out.

And in some circumstances we are well below average. In the global league table for survival rates for cancer we are: cervical cancer 31st out of 62, liver cancer 35th out of 57, brain cancer 44th out of 58, ovarian cancer 45th out of 59, pancreatic cancer 47th out of 56 behind Latvia, Africa and Argentina. We are one the richest countries in the world but our survival rates make us the Cowdenbeath of cancer.

Anecdotally the NHS is best in the world but factually it is average at best, below average for a rich country and eventually anecdotes will catch up with facts and then we might do something about the fact that one in five cancers in the UK are detected in A&E.

That is truly exceptional.

MARK (AS RON): *'Kidneys.'*

We are now on major organ failures. We have been through heart and lungs and now it is…

'…Kidneys. Over 100,000 people die each year of acute kidney illness. Oh what is that twinge in your back, could it be that you have been late night clubbing and left your midriff exposed in haze of day-glo dance fury or is it renal failure.'

Projection on the rear screen of the interior of the Kidney Unit of Hammersmith Hospital.

The Renal Unit at Hammersmith Hospital is not in Hammersmith, it is in East Acton, next to Wormwood Scrubs. It is three floors high.

At the top is the high dependency unit. People who have just had transplants or are in a critical condition. The nurses' station is in the middle of the room. There are no walls. Just glass. The nurses have a 360-degree view of every patient and every monitor attached to them. It is like being at the bridge of a spacecraft.

Below is the ward for infections. If you've had a kidney transplant you are on immunosuppressants to stop the organ being rejected by the body and are therefore prone to infections.

Below that is the Walk-in Assessment centre, which is an A&E just for kidneys. 140 people come through here a day.

Next to that is dialysis, open for three sessions each day, morning, afternoon and 5.30pm–10.30pm. People lie on beds, reading, listening to music, sitting with relatives, many just lie starring into middle distance. Hooked up to the machine that takes their blood, removes the waste and replaces it. It is a quiet room. The occasional hiss from a headphone, the bing of a text arriving and the safe swoosh of the blood pump as it rotates and pumps the blood.

Projection on rear screen: Darren Parsons, Clinical Nephrologist, Hammersmith Hospital, and a small photo of Darren on hospital screen downstage.

Darren Parsons is a Clinical Nephrologist and runs the renal unit.

When I ask him for a photo for the show he says:

'Look there are over 550 people working here, this place is bigger than some district hospitals. Put their photo up.'

I say, *'Do you have one of everyone?'*

'No.'

So this is what he sent me, this, I said to him:

'You do realise it makes you look like one of Hannibal Lecter's victims?'

He says, *'Good. There is not enough fun in medicine.'*

I ask him what he likes about working in the unit?

'It's the contrast. Sometimes it is action stations. You get a donor and you have to do the transplant. One weekend we had three donors and we did the transplants one after the other after the other. And then by comparison I also like the continuity of care. People on dialysis come in three days a week, the average wait for a transplant is three years. And you still need ongoing medical supervision. Each kidney transplant has a half-life of about ten to fifteen

years, so it is not uncommon for people to have two transplants, sometimes three transplants. Some patients will have a lifetime renal career of thirty to forty years. And I like the long-term relationships with the patients.'

I could give you a big statistic but I want to give you a small one, each dialysis session for one person costs £400 and that is three times a week until they get a transplant or die.

And without all of this 3500 people are…pop.

When the NHS was created the founding fathers and mothers thought our health would improve and we would need the NHS less. But in 1948 no one foresaw the advances in medical science and life expectancy.

Now there is a narrative in certain sections of the press, and has been since the NHS came into being, that NHS is a broken left-wing money pit.

And they are kind of right.

Broken?… Well certainly driven to the brink by the spending squeeze.

Is it a left-wing fantasy? … Well it does treat working class people so by press standards the NHS is a Trotskyist plot.

My last interview is with Anita Charlesworth, a health economist. She says that funding the NHS through income tax is the fairest way of doing it cos everyone should contribute – corporations, rich pensioners, those in work, everyone who can should.

Our problem is we have a North American level of tax and expect a Western European level of healthcare and the way that we have lived with that paradox is about to end.

On rear screen a video of an excerpt of the Anita Charlesworth interview is projected.

'Over the last seventy years we have pulled off quite a trick which is the closest we will ever see to 'have cake and eat it'. We have a share of tax out of our overall economy now which isn't that different from seventy years ago…but we have a healthcare spend that has doubled as a share, so we have spent twice as much on healthcare and we seemingly have not had to pay for it through tax, which is fabulous and the way we have done that is that healthcare has taken all the spending from the other things we have cut back and the most obvious big example of that is defence so when we came out of the Second World War we would spend about 10% GDP on defence and

about 3% on healthcare and basically they have reversed.'

The era of low tax is over. She says,

'Some think we can put a slug of money into the NHS and that's it, problem solved, we can walk away, what we have to do is get our heads around the concept that we need to put more money into the NHS year on year. FOREVER.'

And so is it a money pit? Yes it is and we are the money pit, each and everyone of us. Our health is the pit into which we pour the money. Hooofuckingrah!

MARK (AS RON): *'Dementia. Over a 100 different types of dementia. Some say nearly two hundred. There are more types of dementia than there are UKIP councillors.'*

MARK walks to the trolley and washes his hands.

I see the dementia nurses four times during
the course of my residency. This is Jules.

A full-length picture of Jules is projected on the
hospital screen downstage.

When I first meet her I said, '*So you work on*
the dementia ward?'

'*There is not a dementia ward as such because*
dementia is everywhere. People are here for
other reasons, other conditions, they might have
had a fall or heart condition but they have
dementia, they get confused, anxious, some get
aggressive. Our job is to support the clinical staff
and the patients. It is all about patient centred
care, it has to be personalised. One patient kept
shouting at the nurses that they had stolen his
dole money and getting quite aggressive so we

*put some Monopoly money on his bedside under
a paperweight and when he shouted, 'You've
stolen the dole money,' they would point at it and
say, 'There it is,' and he calmed down. Another
patient he would be up all night, sleep in the
day but wandering the wards at night and we
couldn't work out what was going on, then we
spoke to his family and it turned out he used
to be a doorman at a west end nightclub, so we
gave him a clipboard and he used to sign in the
morning shift on the guest list.'*

I am here to meet a woman called Sarah who
has dementia, her two daughters in their mid
forties, have agreed for me to speak to them all.

Sarah has dementia and nothing else wrong
with her but she can become very aggressive
and violent, so her husband sleeps in the car
but parks the car to face the front door and

turns the headlights on, so he can see if she tries to leave the house. And he has COPD Chronic Obstructive Pulmonary Disorder, so he has to take his oxygen with him.

If you want a snap shot of social care in this country it is a husband sleeping in a car with an oxygen tank with the headlamps on the front door to protect his wife.

'In Place of Fear.'

She is in hospital because they have no 'care package'. Before I go in I am told Sarah is originally from Ireland and she came here in her early twenties and that today she is in a good mood, a bit frisky.

Sarah sits up in bed and her daughters by her side.

I walk in,

'Oh, a young one.'

Which isn't a classic symptom of dementia but is in my book.

I say,

'Hi, where are you from, Sarah?'

'I'm from Dublin's fair city, where the girls are so titty…'

Her daughters look at her and tut indulgently.

'I like the dancing. I love the dancing. Down the Palais. I love schwinging the blues. Can you dance? No I'll teach you. Do you know how I meet Tommy, I saw him at the dance and I stuck my foot out. I love the dancing, schwinging the blues.'

Afterwards her daughter says to me,

'Our problem is we need to put her in a care home near us but it costs £995 a week and we cannot afford it.'

A silent video of all three dementia nurses talking together in the hospital is projected on the small hospital screen downstage.

A few weeks later and I am visiting the dementia nurses again, Lucy and Jo are here.

When I first meet Lucy she said,

'I must show you the toy cupboard. People with dementia like soft toys, it calms them down.'

Does the hospital pay for this?

'No, fundraising. Aeish did it.'

*A picture of Aeish is projected on the rear sceen
followed by a picture of the highest part of St
Mary's Hospital*

Aeish is a Northern Irish nurse who recently
left the team for maternity leave. She said, *'I
agreed to do a sponsored abseil to raise money
for the toys. I got all the sponsorship done. I get
to the top and I didn't realise how high it was.
Beneath me are all the bosses and consultants
and management, my employers and I lean off
the edge and shout "FUCKKKKK" and that is
just not like me.'*

I visit the dementia team for the last time and
they are organising a World Cup party for the
patients. Jules says, *'They got a home for Sarah.
We said to the family hold out against social
services, they have to house her. And they did.*

Found a home near the family. Lucy drove them down there.'

How long was she in for?

'Two months. Nothing else wrong with her but nowhere else to go.'

This is the thing, the NHS is not an island, it is a landlocked entity surrounded by the borders of austerity, poverty and social care and that is what walks in through the door.

And that is why a ring-fenced – hypothocated – tax increase for the NHS will never work because the support has to reach out to everyone before they walk in through the doors, we have to raise everyone's health. And if we do not 'take these reasonable measures it is unjust and we are literally taking years off of people's lives.'

As I look at this room of patients in gowns, with hats, surrounded by bunting and flags from across the world. Music playing from the 60s, of table football games, of finger food and non-alcoholic cocktails served from a trolley and the patients getting a little tipsy because they don't know it is non-alcoholic. And Lucy, Jo and Jules, helping with food and singing and playing and smiles. And I have this overwhelming feeling of emotion as I realise I am in the presence of care. And for all the robotics, genomics, biomarkers and nanobots with luck we will all get old, and need care.

And when I get old these are the people I want.

I have spent the whole afternoon with Ron running through the possible scenarios of my demise.

MARK (AS RON): *'Well I think I covered it. You know this has really cheered me up. I was feeling down before I came here. You know what we have forgotten? Auto erotic asphyx…'*

No Ron, we're fine.

'You know all this reminds me of that old joke, there are only two certainties in life. Death and taxes. The only choice we have is how much do you want to pay of one to stave off the other for as long possible. How much do you want to pay?'

What I love about the NHS is that for all its science and technology it is held together by faith. By the goodwill of the people who work here and they work harder and longer to hold it together because of a very unfashionable concept, duty. Public Service. And a sense of public service can only exist in a body that works for the greater good of everyone. And you will never get that with private profit.

LX: blackout.

SFX: John Coltrane – 'Favourite Things'.

Video of MARK walking up ramp and into Lisson Grove Health Centre.

WWW.OBERONBOOKS.COM

Follow us on www.twitter.com/@oberonbooks
& www.facebook.com/OberonBooksLondon